CLEAN EATING

By Debi L. Smith

ISBN-13: 978-1973940548
ISBN-10: 197394054X

Contact the Author

Facebook: @Debi L. Smith

CONTENTS

ACKNOWLEDGMENTS i

1 START SMALL 1

2 CHANGE YOUR DIET 5

3 COOKING 10

4 RECIPES 16

5 DOING IT ON A BUDGET 29

6 NO TIME FOR COOKING 33

7 EATING OUT 37

8 CRAVINGS 40

9 EXERCISE 43

10 WORKOUT 46

11 COMMITMENT 50

12 BE KIND TO YOURSELF 54

My Story 59

ACKNOWLEDGMENTS

I would like to dedicate this book to Eileen who gave me the idea of reaching others, and Abman who encouraged me to actually write a book, and in loving memory of *my little Ronan*.

I am also deeply grateful to Kay Sheppard, whose understanding of food addiction and work in the field saved my life.

1

START SMALL

"The journey of a thousand miles begins with a single step." Lao TZU

So, just begin. Drink a little more WATER, get a little more SLEEP, move a little more (take the stairs, park further away, walk to Starbucks or local errands, or even the mailbox to start). Add fresh fruits and vegetables to your diet (starting wherever you are). It is NOT about calories and portion control; it's about WHAT you eat and when you eat it. These very simple changes will change your life; they will improve your energy level, your mood, and your skin, not to mention the impact on general health (lowering risk of cancer and other diseases as well as the common cold). You will FEEL better and LOOK better.

I feel better in my late forties than I ever did in my

twenties and thirties. My eyes are brighter, my skin is clearer, my unruly naturally curly hair is the best it's ever looked, and my body is lean and strong in ways that I'm not sure it ever was before. I am happier and healthier as well as more productive. Food has, quite literally, become fuel, rather than a drug; it feeds me and gives me energy, rather than tearing me down emotionally and physically. That energy is also a natural, healthy one that is a byproduct of clean living rather than chemicals like caffeine and sugar.

So, when it comes to food use CLEAN ingredients (no preservatives, steroids, or anything pre-marinated or seasoned). I understand we can't all afford organic; I myself do not buy all organic but at least start with real, whole food. Then, use olive oil, coconut oil, nut oils, fresh whole herbs and spices, garlic, and lemon. Food will taste better, promote better health, and cause significantly fewer cravings (there will be a whole chapter devoted to this). When it comes to produce, ADD it to your diet, don't starve yourself trying to live off of it. Instead, choose healthy proteins and starches (fish, chicken, turkey, good eggs, tofu, beans, edamame, brown rice, wild rice, and sweet potatoes).

When you eat out, make better choices (health food stores and restaurants, fish houses, grills, rotisserie's etc.) and ask for brown rice and no sauce and lots of veggies. Everything tastes wonderful with olive oil, fresh garlic, sea salt (or kosher salt) and pepper so order it prepared that way - even if it's a burger or steak, at least have it prepared that way with no bread, cheese, or sauces.

And, don't forget water and sleep. Drinking enough WATER is one of the very best things you can do for yourself. It has so many health benefits. Also, research suggests that thirst feels very much like hunger to the body, and is frequently mistaken for hunger so, if you're not drinking enough water, you may be overeating at mealtime or snacking in between meals because you feel hungry. Test it for yourself; next time you feel hungry, between meals, try drinking a couple glasses of water and waiting just a few minutes. In fact, even if it is mealtime, when you are perhaps waiting for your order, drink a full glass of water instead of eyeing the bread or chips on the table.

Sadly, SLEEP is so undervalued in our society. In fact, it seems like we are forever looking for new ways to avoid it. All those energy drinks, caffeine pills, sodas, coffee, etc. etc., that are designed to give us a boost, have become so popular. I have never slept better, or felt better, since I got off of it all. I was so physically addicted that the detox was pretty awful but I feel amazing now. I try to get enough sleep regularly (7-8 hours a night) but I also listen to my body. If I'm tired, I rest and I've become a big fan of naps, even short *power* naps. Even if I've gotten a good night's sleep, if I feel tired, I take a nap or go to bed a little earlier or take a night off to relax. I find that sometimes it's just rest my body craves rather than sleep. I try to give it both.

So, again, start small, from wherever you are, but start! Don't put it off another day. You can't afford to wait for the right set of circumstances because there is no such thing. Or, worse yet is waiting until you feel like it... inspired, ready, etc. Action always precedes feeling, in my experience. If you take the right action you will begin to feel better. If you wait to feel, you may never get there because you haven't taken the right actions. Someone once told me that the good news about this spiritual law is that you can feel just as crummy, negative, resistant, etc. as a person can and, as long as you take the right action, you will get the desired results. In fact, if my experience means anything at all, you will get the results whether you like it or not, which you will certainly come to appreciate.

2

CHANGE YOUR DIET

Forbes says, "If you are one of the 100 million American's trying to lose weight, here's a hot tip: Don't go on a diet".

Diets don't work. Personally, I am more impressed with visible results than written statistics but this is a pretty staggering one and many sources agree. *95% of diets fail and most will regain their lost weight in 1-5 years.* Despite an estimated $65 billion spent on various weight loss efforts, 69.2% of American's over 20 are overweight. *Diets do not lead to sustained weight loss*. UCLA researchers reported in the journal of the American Psychological Association. The most comprehensive and rigorous analysis of diet studies, analyzing 31 long-term studies, concluded that, *the majority of people regained all the weight, plus more*. Their evidence also suggests that repeatedly losing and gaining weight is linked to cardiovascular disease, stroke, diabetes and altered immune function. Scary stuff if you ask me.

Rather than going on a diet, change your diet. Most of us have done our share of yoyo dieting and discovered, for ourselves, that they are temporary at best. Lifetime changes will produce lifetime results. I myself have tried many diets and programs (some more than once), read so many books, and purchased expensive products designed to replace meals, and oh my goodness SO many protein bars, and although I have sometimes lost weight I have never felt free from food cravings and I have always gained the weight back eventually. It's incredibly painful emotionally and physically. Research suggests that dieting may be harder on your body than being overweight is. Think about that. Dieting is a trauma to the body.

The whole diet craze can be so enticing, particularly when there are beautiful, fit people promoting them. Then, there are the expensive programs, and sadly even surgery, but you can't buy freedom; there's simply no way to bypass the hard work and sometimes painfully slow results. The good news is that slow and steady progress seems to be the recipe for long-lasting results whereas those quick fixes seem to be lost just as quickly. Remember, I have been doing this since Easter of 2008 and am more fit today than ever before. Believe it or not, I lost two more pants sizes in the last couple of years, in my late forties, post-menopause, when other women are gaining no matter what they do.

Start by cutting out junk food; it's garbage and quite literally poisonous. Caffeine is a stimulant and stimulates the appetite so if you can cut it out or even cut back it will help your cause. Try adding fruit (a relatively small apple, orange, pear, etc.) to your breakfast and vegetables (a large helping) to lunch and dinner. Produce has all kinds of wonderful health benefits, plus it will round out your meals, fill you up, and produce fewer cravings. It also adds color and looks beautiful on your plate. My food is more visually, and I imagine psychologically, appealing than ever.

Find good, healthy food and recipes you find delicious. Fall in love with food and try everything - even if you used to hate it because food and taste buds can be funny that way. Try them cooked, raw, and prepared different ways. If you don't like something this month, try it again next month. Some of my very favorite foods today are among those I hated growing up and, in some cases, well into adulthood.

I absolutely love Brussels sprouts, for instance, and I have a vivid childhood memory of being up quite late on a school night because I wasn't allowed to leave the dinner table until I ate them. I also thought tomatoes were gross well into adulthood and today they are one of my very favorites; I eat them raw, cooked, sliced and salted, or just popped in my mouth when it comes to the little sweet ones. Onions were perhaps the worst and today there is nothing that isn't made better with onions (white, red, green, raw and cooked). Funny how things change.

In fact, my taste buds are still changing years into eating this way. It's kind of incredible, as a matter of fact. Two years ago, I hated cooked carrots and now I really enjoy them in certain things. I also just fell in love with sweet potatoes this year, because of a sweet potato dish that a friend turned me on to and will be sure to share the recipe (in Chapter 4). Hope you enjoy it as well!

I haven't had wheat, flour, or sugar since Easter of 2008. It has changed my weight, my skin, my mood, and energy level. I'm sure that I am more enthusiastic about exercise and working out because of it as well. Just to be clear, I don't do any alternative, chemical, fake, or *natural* sugars either - ever. So, no honey, guava, Equal, Stevia, etc. etc. And, no diet sodas or Starbucks flavored anything (including almond or soy milk). Ironically, *sugar free* products are almost always jampacked full of these fake sugars in order to make them taste better so steer clear of them.

I get my *sugar* and sweet flavor from the fresh fruit in my diet, which is my very favorite thing today, and coconut oil (which I love on my pancakes). For whatever reason, I have found that although very good for you, most brands are quite bland. Fortunately, I was encouraged to try Nutiva and I have not bought anything else since. It is available online and I buy it locally at

Target, Sprouts, and Mother's Market & Kitchen.

So, to sum up, do away with traditional dieting - that mentality is deadly - and change your diet. Start small but start today. Eliminate something that's no good for you and add something wonderfully delicious and healthy. DON'T skip breakfast. Fuel your body with nutritious food. Bring a healthy lunch with you, if there are no healthy choices available. I work for the school district and, sadly, there is nothing available at school that I would eat. Choose a healthy restaurant, even if it's fast food.

Personally, I do not recommend snacking - even healthy snacks - it is an unhealthy practice deeply engrained in many of us. If you are feeding your body what it needs at meal time, there will be no need for snacking. Try drinking water in between meals instead; it's so good for you! Also, if you're really having trouble making it to mealtime (perhaps waiting on your food, for instance) eat some raw veggies and subtract them from your meal. Consider incorporating a salad even if you were planning on having a different vegetable.

3

COOKING

John Hopkins Center for a Livable Future says that findings suggest that home cooking is a main ingredient in healthier eating.

Cooking at home has so many health benefits. Selecting and purchasing your own ingredients controls the quality of the food you cook, eat, and serve the people you love. Preparing it yourself allows you to use healthier ingredients and bypass all the preservatives and processing that's unnecessary with real, fresh, food. Their research shows that home cooking leads to better health, greater weight loss, and saving money in the long run.

So, plan, prep, and shop for clean eating. Choose your markets and your staples. I use a club store, a health food store, a farmer's type market, as well as the more traditional supermarkets for a couple items. I've learned where I can get good eggs, produce, meat, seafood, etc. at the best prices. Make and use a LIST! I have one for each store with all the items available listed.

Here is a glimpse of my staples:

Old Bay Seasoning

Newman's Own Oil & Vinegar Dressing

*** I keep a bottle in my car**

Bragg's Amino Acids

Clean Mustard (Yellow & Dijon)

Fresh Minced Garlic

*** My dollar store sells it :)**

Sea Salt or Kosher Salt (not iodized)

Black Pepper

Oat Bran

Oatmeal (no quick, instant, or flavored)

Greek Yogurt (nonfat & unflavored - Fage is my favorite)

Buttermilk (Trader Joe's is cheap if you have one)

Whole Herbs & Spices (Cumin, Smoked Paprika, Thyme, Red Pepper Flakes, Cilantro, Parsley, Chives, Oregano, Dry Mustard, Cayenne Pepper, Sage, Cinnamon, Chili Powder, Onion Powder, Clean Italian Seasoning)

Blueberries

Strawberries

Grapefruit

Oranges

Apples

Pears

Nut Oil (Walnut is relatively inexpensive and my personal favorite)

Olive Oil

Coconut Oil (Nutiva is my favorite and very sweet)

Brussels Sprouts

Sweet Potatoes

Red Onions

White Onions

Frozen Brown Rice

Raw Brown Rice

Canned Tomatoes

Tomato Sauce

Tomato Paste

Canned Green Beans

Lemons (Meyer are especially yummy)

Fresh Tomatoes (I love the little sweet ones)

Cucumbers (I prefer the Persian)

Bag of Raw Carrots

Clean Pizza Sauce (Muir Glen Organic is delicious)

Clean Extra Firm Tofu (I use Wild Woods in the plastic wrap)

Eggs (use good eggs - pay for them - it's worth it - Happy Eggs are the best I've found)

Clean Soymilk (soybeans and water only - Trader Joe's

brand is cheap if you have one)

Non-Fat Milk Powder (Bob's Red Mill or Carnation)

*** Bob's is much better but more expensive**

Butter (grass fed and unsalted)

Fish (I eat a lot of Salmon and Tilapia)

Sparkling Water (non-flavored)

If finances are limited, start with a short list. You may even have some of these items in your cupboards already. Collect things when they are on sale. I've gotten fresh minced garlic at a dollar store and it was wonderful. I could live on eggs, oat bran, milk powder, buttermilk, fresh produce, walnut oil, the Newman's salad dressing, fresh garlic, sea salt, pepper, brown rice or potatoes, and fish for quite a while. If fish is not within your budget, replace it with chicken, eggs, and ground turkey.

I realize that not all of us enjoy cooking - I know I didn't - but, falling in love with your wonderful, home-cooked meals will help. Truth be told, I probably love eating what I prepare far more than actually cooking it. I have really come to enjoy the planning; I am always thinking about what I'm going to have for my next meal, over the weekend, or for a special occasion. So, be creative and daydream a little.

Also, keep in mind, cooking doesn't have to be elaborate. Buy simple ingredients and make simple dishes. I take advantage of a lot of prepped options at the market. It saves me so much time and if you go to the right stores it's not even expensive. Try canned vegetables in recipes that call for fresh; frequently, you can't tell the difference by the time it's done. You will get a feel for how to save yourself time and money and most of us appreciate that.

Cooking is key but don't let it be a deal breaker. It can be done at your pace, starting wherever you are. Perhaps you can get your spouse or children involved. They may not have a problem with food or weight but clean, healthy cooking and eating is ideal for everyone's health. At one point, I had two girlfriends that were so interested in eating this way, having watched me have the experience I'd had, that we would have cooking dates. They would come over and the three of us would cook together, making quite a mess but, having a great time and ending up with some wonderful home-cooked meals. Sometimes, we cooked individually, choosing three different dishes, and then split them up so that we had more variety, which was really nice. Thank you Julie and Victoria!

So, have fun with friends or family, or experimenting on your own, but, start cooking!

4

RECIPES

Collect recipes and then modify and recreate as much as necessary. I have several wonderful recipes that I only had to delete one ingredient or change white rice to brown. Many recipes add a small amount of sugar, even many you wouldn't expect to, so I just don't add it. Consider old family recipes, search the internet, use health magazines and recipe books. There are so many sources.

I have several favorite recipes I'd like to share; perhaps you will enjoy some of them as well and hopefully they will inspire you to find and make your own. I will include some options for breakfast, lunch and dinner (which are interchangeable), as well as the kind of thing I have for my evening snack. They will be complete meal options that I eat in one sitting.

Here are a couple of my favorite breakfasts:

Blueberry Loaf:

* I got this recipe from a friend but I believe it originally came from Kay Sheppard's, cook book, *Absolutely Abstinent!* (which I own, and highly recommend, if you can afford it).

Thank you, Kay!

2 eggs

1/2 cup oat bran

1/3 cup milk powder

6 oz. blueberries (fresh or frozen)

* fresh is so much better!

Mix ingredients (do not add water to the milk powder or mixture) & transfer to a sprayed Pyrex loaf pan. It will only be perhaps an inch high but should fill the entire pan. Cook at 350 degrees for approximately 25 minutes & eat fresh, right out of the oven. You can batch cook these and even freeze if necessary for traveling.

Buttermilk Pancakes:

2 eggs

1/2 cup oat bran

1 cup buttermilk

Mix ingredients to make the batter. You will find that it is too thin but just put it in the fridge for a bit before cooking and then proceed like you would with any other pancake batter. I add 6 oz. of fruit to make it a full breakfast. You can put berries in the batter or add any fruit of your choice on the side. Pancakes with fresh strawberries is one of my very favorite breakfasts. I top the pancakes with a bit of coconut or walnut oil. I especially love the walnut oil with these.

Another option is to use 1/2 cup of buttermilk (which is plenty) and cover them in 1/3 cup of Greek yogurt and fresh fruit. You might want to experiment with different kinds of fruit or use cinnamon, either in the batter or sprinkled on top. I especially love cinnamon with apples. I sometimes use 1/2 cup of buttermilk and eat one light string cheese for the rest of the dairy serving.

Greek Yogurt Pancakes:

2 eggs

1/2 cup oat bran

3/4 cup Greek yogurt (non-fat, unflavored)

This batter will be thick and creamy and give a little different taste and texture to your pancakes. Again, I add 6 oz. of fruit. I make blueberry pancakes occasionally, but actually prefer fresh fruit on the side. You can also crush fresh berries on top almost like a jelly. I especially love the coconut oil on these.

Homemade Turkey Sausage:

1/3 lb. ground turkey (this is essentially the equivalent of 4 oz. cooked or 2 eggs)

Add:

1/4 tsp. sea salt

1/2 tsp. pepper

1/2 tsp. smoked paprika

1/2 tsp. dry mustard

1/4 tsp. chili pepper flakes

* Play with the spices to suit your taste; you may like your sausage a bit saltier or spicier, for instance. Add cayenne for hot sausage.

Blend like meatloaf and make small patties out of the mixture. To make a complete breakfast, you can add a clean grain or starch, dairy or 1/2 protein, and fruit. I enjoy having an egg (1/2 protein) with it along with oatmeal (1 cup) covered in diced apples and cinnamon.

The sausage is also great for work lunches. You can add a clean starch or grain like potatoes, brown rice, or maybe clean (& fat free) refried beans, and veggies to make it into a full meal. Amy's brand has a canned lentil soup in low sodium that I love that goes nicely with these too.

You can also add a clean pasta sauce, crumble the meat, and make spaghetti using spaghetti squash as your starch. You will find that ground turkey, like chicken, is very versatile; you just have to get creative so have fun with it.

* Please note: If you can't tolerate the oat bran based breakfasts initially, don't worry. I hated them the first few times I tried them but, taste buds change once sugar is eliminated. They are my very favorites today. The fresh blueberry loaf is heavenly and, honestly, I recall thinking it was bland and dry.

The following are a couple of my favorite lunches/dinners:

Columbian Chicken:

* This is an old Columbian family recipe; thank you, Gina!

4 oz. cooked chicken (perhaps shredded pieces from a whole chicken done in the crockpot)

1 cup diced tomatoes (canned is fine)

1 cup diced onions

1 cup green beans (canned is fine)

1/3 cup brown rice (uncooked)

chicken broth (perhaps from the chicken/crockpot)

Sautee the vegetables, add the chicken, and 1 cup of broth and 1 cup of water to start, adding what you need to as you go. Bring to a boil and add the rice. Cook on medium to medium high until the rice is done. This dish is a little work but so flavorful and one of my all-time favorites. I cook four at a time, using all the burners on my stove.

Sweet Potato Dish:

This is a new favorite & absolutely delicious!

10 oz. sweet potato (peeled and diced)

1 cup red onion (peeled and diced)

1 tbsp. Dijon mustard

1 tsp. thyme

1/2 tsp. salt

1/2 tsp. pepper

Mix ingredients and transfer to a sprayed oven safe dish and cook at 450 degrees for approximately 45 minutes. Spray and stir half way through for best results. I love this dish with fish and Brussels sprouts which makes it a full meal. So, here are two easy recipes for them :)

Fish:

I eat a lot of salmon and tilapia but there are so many other varieties that are very nice too - try them all!

Heavily coat both sides in Old Bay Seasoning and cook in a greased pan on med high heat. Timing varies quite a bit but it won't take long; just brown both sides and make sure it's not raw in the middle. This method is so quick and easy and perfect every time.

Alternatively, replace the Old Bay with a little fresh garlic and sea salt and use the same cooking method.

Brussels Sprouts:

I cut them in half and steam them for just a couple of minutes (2-5 minutes depending on amount and size) before cooking. Then I throw them in a greased pan on medium high heat, adding lemon (Meyer lemons are my favorite but can be harder to find and are much more expensive) and salt and pepper, and cook until browned.

Quick *fried* rice is an alternative to the sweet potato dish and has become one of my favorites.

Quick *Fried* Rice

1 cup brown rice

1 tsp. Bragg's Amino Acids

green onions (to taste)

Grease pan with olive oil and cook rice and green onions on medium high heat. This is very easy and fast and quite tasty. If you like, you can also put two beaten eggs in it as your protein and just add some veggies for a full meal.

Any onions will work, of course, and I recently discovered that leftover chicken, onions, and brown rice sautéed in chicken broth is really delicious.

Potato Skins:

These are very fast and easy! Microwave potatoes, scoop out some of the inside (which I save for mashed potatoes), spray both sides with cooking spray, and add salt and pepper before putting in the broiler for maybe three minutes on each side. I use 8 ounces for a meal serving. You can add beans, meat and veggies for a more traditional potato skin, but will want to adjust for the starch. If you add 1/2 cup of beans just use 4 oz. of potato. It is possible to make this an entire meal.

* And speaking of mashed potatoes :)

Mashed Potatoes:

Take 10 oz. of cooked and peeled, or unpeeled potatoes. Add 1/4 cup of soy milk, and salt and pepper. These take 5 minutes if you've already got the potato saved and not much longer even if you don't. They are very tasty and satisfying.

Mexican Fiesta:

1/3 lb. ground meat (I recommend grass fed beef or turkey)

1 cup cooked brown rice

1 cup diced onion

1 cup tomato sauce

1 tsp. tomato paste

1/2 tsp. cumin

1/4 tsp. chili powder

1/4 tsp. pepper

Cook meat and onion with the cumin. Then, drain. Add the tomato sauce, tomato paste, chili powder, pepper, and one cup of water. Cook on medium for a few minutes and then simmer as long as possible. The longer it cooks the more flavorful it will be; I like to do it while I'm doing laundry. Add the rice at the end and eat or store. This dish is particularly good leftover. I also always cook two or three servings at a time and like to use it for work lunches.

Omelette:

I have always loved breakfast for dinner so here is a recipe for an omelette that is wonderful with the sweet potato dish or even clean, fat-free, refried beans (1 cup).

2 eggs

2-3 cups of spinach

1/2 cup of red onion (diced)

2-3 small mushrooms

1/4 tsp. salt

1/4 tsp. pepper

You can play with the vegetable amounts or experiment with different choices but this is so fast and easy and quite good. I cook the veggies in a greased pan on medium high heat and then pour the beaten eggs over them adding the salt and pepper. You can add fresh sliced tomatoes on top. Although visually appealing, I found it a little wet for my taste :) Remember, add the sweet potato dish or beans to make a full meal. Potato skins might go nicely as well.

* Just as breakfast is wonderful for dinner, I have enjoyed several dinner protein options for breakfast. Don't hesitate to try it all; I have had salmon for breakfast and loved it. I am careful to have fruit with my breakfast and vegetables with my lunch but just about everything else is interchangeable.

Salsa Marinated Ground Turkey Lettuce Wrapped Tacos:

1/3 lb. ground turkey

1 cup clean salsa (veggies, spices, and olive oil only)

lettuce (or cabbage) leaves

1 cup raw veggies on the side

I crumble one of the ground turkey patties (5.5 oz.) into a pan and cook slowly in the salsa. Then, I scoop the mixture into two lettuce leaves and have some kind of fresh vegetable on the side. I add a cup of clean fat-free refried beans to make it a full meal. You can eat the beans on the side or scoop them into the tacos as well.

* This is a seriously inexpensive meal that I especially love to have during the summer. If you buy the ingredients when they're on sale, you can eat or feed your entire family for almost nothing. I have gotten refried beans for 59 cents a can and salsa for as little as two dollars and usually buy the turkey at Costco but occasionally it's even cheaper on sale at the market.

I also love the Italian Casserole recipe found in Kay's cookbook. It is delicious leftover, just warmed up in the microwave. I usually make three at a time because that's what I can fit in the oven.

Here are a couple of my favorite evening snacks:

Please note: I have a very bad habit of calling it my snack but this is really more of a metabolic 1/2 meal to control blood sugar overnight.

1/2 protein (1 egg for instance or leftover meat - 2 oz. cooked - work great) and 6 oz. fresh fruit

* I have fallen in love with some strange combinations :)

3/4 cup Greek yogurt (non-fat, unflavored only)

6 oz. fresh fruit

1 cup soymilk (soybeans and water only) and 6 oz. fresh or frozen fruit)

* Use blender to make smoothie

I also like to freeze smoothies during the summer & eat them like frozen yogurt or ice cream. You can also make popsicles.

* While cheese is probably not the best option, one of my very favorites is:

2 light string cheese and 6 oz. fresh fruit (I especially love apples, pears, and strawberries with cheese)

So, again, be creative. Recipes can be nothing more than a starting place. If you hate blueberries, for instance, but the loaf sounds delicious, try another fruit. Or, try it with vegetables for lunch or dinner. My girlfriend loved making them with canned pumpkin and shredded carrots and cinnamon. I've discovered that the sugar free pizza sauce makes just about anything pretty wonderful. Especially with sautéed onions and sweet peppers. So, have fun with it.

One secret I'll share: Even when on a budget, I refuse to eat anything I really don't like, unless it's a bona fide emergency. So, don't worry if you have more disasters than successes at first; toss them and try again.

5

DOING IT ON A BUDGET

Contrary to popular belief, it is not more expensive to eat healthy or to eat in rather than out. "Cooking at home is cheaper than eating out - always, and by a wide margin." The Boston Globe printed and thoroughly debunked a claim to the contrary.

You absolutely can afford to eat healthy. Please don't let finances keep you from changing your life, and perhaps saving it. Raw brown rice and beans are super cheap and versatile. Buy some herbs and spices at your local dollar store. As I mentioned, I even found minced garlic! Collect canned goods when they are on sale. I sometimes get them as cheap as 59 cents a can.

I eat a lot of fish which is so good for you but it isn't always the best option when living on a budget. I buy 5% ground turkey burgers at our local Costco; a bag of twelve is $10.99 and each patty is a perfect protein for any meal. Buy whole chickens when they are ridiculously cheap; there is so much you can do with them. Use more onion (white, red, and green). I also buy a box of canned green beans at Costco which is very inexpensive. They have diced tomatoes as well. There are so many things you can do with chicken, onions, tomatoes and rice. Don't forget the Columbian Chicken!

If you aren't a member of your local club/discount store, chances are that one (or more) of your family members or friends are and would be happy to have you join them, perhaps once a month, or even just pick up one or two items for you when they are there. Be resourceful.

I save a fortune doing all the above. It's not very often that I shop for a particular recipe; I keep things on hand and perhaps pick up one or two fresh ingredients I need. Find a source for cheap produce and then buy whatever is on sale to save even more.

I just got 6 oz. packages of fresh blackberries for eighty-eight cents apiece! I frequently get grapefruit on sale, three for a dollar, and oranges are sometimes two pounds for a dollar. Potatoes and red onion are always economical and you can do so much with them.

Jenny-O brand has a sweet turkey sausage that is totally clean and very tasty. The price in my local markets varies from $4.99 to $6.49 a package but I have gotten them on sale for $3.99 a number of times. They cook up very quickly and are great left over for work lunches or even to use as a breakfast protein or evening snack in a pinch.

Doctor up brown rice with Bragg's Amino Acids and green onions. Bragg's is inexpensive and goes a long way and onions are super cheap. Add some additional veggies and a clean protein (perhaps the Jenny-O turkey sausage sliced up) and you have a full meal. You can buy raw rice very inexpensively and cook in bulk (and even freeze) or you can buy it fully cooked (in the freezer section) but just make sure it's nothing but rice and water.

If you have, or can get or borrow, an inexpensive slow cooker you can save so much money and time. Soups and stews can be made overnight and provide full meals for at home as well as for work lunches. You can also throw in whole chickens overnight and make Columbian chicken, and other chicken based dishes, or soup.

Eventually, eating this way will become second nature and you will come up with many new ways to save money, as well as creative ways to do more with the food you buy and cook. Although I don't always, I have spent just a couple of hours on a Saturday or Sunday cooking and, in addition to making myself a nice meal to eat then, ended up with enough food for the entire work week and several evening dinners and snacks very inexpensively.

So, please, believe me when I say: You can afford to eat

healthy. You can afford to feed your family healthy food. You can afford to change your health and your life.

6

NO TIME FOR COOKING

Eating out, like so many other things, always seems like the faster option but be sure you consider all the factors. You can go grocery shopping once and eat in all week where as you are likely to be traveling for every meal out. Also, there is the wait to order or be seated, and paying is often a separate wait, whether eating at a fast food, take out, or dine in restaurant. Even the convenient drive through options often take longer than parking and going in.

Starbucks is an excellent example. Consider the difference between making your own coffee at home, or at work for that matter, and going to Starbucks for every cup; full service is not only costly but so time consuming. Eating out is much the same no matter how you do it.
Bottom line, you are going to spend time ordering, paying, and waiting for the food. Then, you will perhaps

travel to someplace else to eat it.

Although I do most of my own cooking and recommend it, I understand there are times where it seems there just isn't enough time in the day. One of the things that has saved me is batch cooking and food prep. When I take time to make myself a nice dinner I try to cook enough for one or two work lunches as well.

Frequently, over the weekend, I will cook enough of one or two things for the entire work week. When I make Columbian Chicken, for instance, I usually make at least four at a time. It is one of my favorite meals for work lunch, or leftovers in general.

When it comes to fresh vegetables, I use a lot of mini sweet tomatoes which don't require anything but purchase and I always look for sales. Others, that do require a bit of prep, I portion out and have them ready to go in the fridge in storage bags. I eat two full cups of vegetable with each meal (whether within a dish or fresh on the side).

I like to have my work lunches ready for the week; it makes me feel more comfortable about my food. Also, when you know you're going to have a particularly hectic week, give yourself a break and plan to use some of the quickest and easiest recipes. Good food doesn't have to be elaborate.

Have frozen brown rice on hand (you can buy it fully

cooked, in the frozen section). Use the Bragg's Amino Acids and onions to doctor it up, as mentioned in the previous chapter. Again, add some additional veggies and a clean protein (remember, eggs work just fine) and you have a full meal. The Jenny-O turkey sausage cooks very quickly and freezes nicely. It's always nice when you can save money and time.

One of the things that I have learned over time is that recipe times aren't always the best way to determine what I have time for. Some require very little prep and then are just cooked in the oven for a period of time. So, if you are going to be home anyways, don't be afraid of 45 minutes, or even hour plus recipes. Try them when you're home cleaning house, doing laundry, or the kid's homework, etc. etc.

My blueberry loaf takes 30 minutes with prep time but it only takes a few minutes to get it in the oven. I take a bath and get ready for work, while it's cooking. You can also put a whole chicken in the crockpot overnight or sometime over the weekend.

I often cook Columbian Chicken, for instance, in stages. First, I get the chicken cooked in the crockpot. Then, I store the fresh broth in a separate container. When I have time, I shred up the chicken and portion it out (4 oz. per dish/meal) and just throw it in storage bags, if I'm not ready to cook. It might be a day, or two, before I cook the actual dish and that's just fine.

Again, cooking doesn't have to be elaborate. You can cook up some ground meat and then portion it out (I have been taught to use 4 oz. for women and 6 oz. for men) adding canned beans, tomatoes, paste, and yummy spices to make a quick chili. I just cooked a whole chicken in the slow cooker overnight, removed it & threw it in a storage bag, and then cooked two large platters of prepped vegetables and small red potatoes (I picked up at the market) in the chicken broth. It smells amazing! I'm going to make chicken soup with it using the red potatoes for one or two servings and then brown rice for the rest. So, simple but hearty and comforting, particularly during the winter months.

7

EATING OUT

Food network says, "You can eat out and still eat healthy food." In fact, there are more healthy options than ever but there are also many healthy sounding choices that are "diet bombs," so don't assume that, because it's on the light menu, it must be healthy.

Eating out can be tricky, especially in the beginning, but if you're able and willing to be assertive about your special needs it can be done. Fish houses, and steak houses are often pretty accommodating, and two of my very favorites. Call ahead and confirm that they have protein options that are not pre-seasoned or marinated and ask if they can prepare them with olive oil, fresh garlic, and sea or kosher salt. As I mentioned in the beginning, everything is wonderful prepared that way. As long as they have a baked potato and salad or clean vegetable option, you've got a wonderful, full meal.

There are also several health-conscious grills where you can get chicken or fish, vegetables, and brown rice (although you may have to request it and pay a bit extra). I have an Asian grill and a rotisserie chicken place I love. There is even a Chinese place that delivers that has one thing I can have (special ordered, of course). My favorite Mexican place prepares spicy carrots and cauliflower every day, and I get some to go regularly to use as my vegetable for work lunches, and buy party platters of it for casual social events.

If you're really desperate, there are even some fast food options that I trust. I have eaten at Chipotle, El Pollo Loco, and Wendy's, for instance. They are not my favorites and far more difficult to ensure I get the right amounts to control my blood sugar but I have done all three more than once. There are only two protein choices at Chipotle that don't have sugar in them and the pinto beans are cooked with bacon so I get the black or just stick to the brown rice; I eat the chicken, vegetables, and pinto beans at El Pollo Loco; and at Wendy's I just do plain hamburger patties (degreasing as much as possible), a plain baked potato, and a side salad (always asking for no cheese, croutons, etc.)

The hardest part, and perhaps most important for me, has been being willing to tell my friends and family what my needs are in this area. Most of my closest loved ones have been very supportive but some still don't understand and even pick on me a little. I had to decide what was more important, and, for me, there was no question it was my abstinence, health, and sanity. So, I don't hesitate to tell people upfront, ask questions, call ahead, determine whether I can eat there safely, or perhaps bring some food with me to supplement. I bring my own salad dressing, for instance, just about everywhere I go. I actually have a bottle in my car, since it doesn't need to be refrigerated.

So, to sum up, eating out clean can absolutely be done but you will have to take some personal responsibility for your health and needs. If asking for what you need when ordering feels like too much, ask for help. Lean on those that love and support you. I have learned to refer to my food issues as food allergies, which as it turns out is pretty accurate. Restaurants are becoming more and more sensitive and understanding, when it comes to food allergies, and many are very accommodating.

8

CRAVINGS

"Sugar is eight times more addictive than cocaine," says a recent study by Dr. Nicole Avena, a highly respected addiction scientist. She claims that pizza is the most addictive food by far due to the hidden sugar contained in just one slice. The tomato sauce, for instance, can have more sugar than a few Oreos.

As promised, I want to talk just a little about food cravings. Although not at all my area of expertise, I do have a ton of experience and just want to share that it's not weakness or gluttony - it's chemical! I don't pretend to understand the science behind it but the cravings for certain foods, or more food, seem to be produced by certain foods. I have eliminated them from my diet and no longer have food cravings. I enjoy my food very much and look forward to mealtime but I don't crave, anything, ever.

For some people, trying to have one cookie or a small slice of cake or just a few chips is like an alcoholic trying to have one drink. I am one of those people so I don't do it anymore. Getting off sugar, junk food, and caffeine can be incredibly difficult and painful (emotionally and physically) but once it's out of your system you can be free. I can honestly say that I no longer miss them either. It was difficult in the beginning but today it doesn't bother me at all. It no longer looks or smells so good and doesn't call to me like it once did.

Here is a list of things I have eliminated from my diet: sugar, wheat, flour, bananas, mango, grapes, cherries, avocado, corn, nuts (nut oils are fine). So, I never eat bread, buns, or tortillas, nor do I ever put cheese on or in anything anymore, or dip anything in ketchup, barbecue sauce, or chip dip. I do love clean humus and will eat raw carrots and celery sticks with it. I have also found a clean mayonnaise (at our local Trader Joes) that I love to make chicken salad with. I try not to eat things that remind me of my favorite junk foods and instead come up with new healthy favorites.

Believe me, I know it sounds crazy but, I eat better than I have in my entire life. I have a steak dinner with baked potato and salad at least once a month at a local steak house. I frequently eat at a local fish house and have fish, baked potato, and salad. Occasionally, I will even have a burger (with no bun, cheese, or sauce of course). I regularly make grilled shrimp, with my sweet potato dish and Brussels sprouts at home. Not to mention, fresh blueberry loaves and pancakes most every morning.

So, if you struggle with cravings, you made need to eliminate certain things from your diet as well, permanently, if you want the results to be permanent. Detox can be brutal but, once complete, you will have an all new experience around food and feel like a different person - a happier, healthier person!

9

EXERCISE

"Less than 5% of adults participate in 30 minutes of physical activity each day; only one in three adults receive the recommended amount of physical activity each week," says the President's Council on Fitness, Sports and Nutrition.

Again, start small but you have to start (wherever you are) so MOVE - stand instead of sit, use the stairs instead of the elevator, walk instead of drive, and if your health allows, workout! Walking and hiking are wonderful and great for your heart and general health but workouts will change your body. Much like with food, try everything (walking, bicycling, hiking, swimming, roller skating, a sport, a dance class, a workout video, a class at the gym or local YMCA).

I was fortunate enough to workout with personal

trainers in the beginning and it is truly priceless. Having said that, I understand that it is very expensive. A new gym opened in my area and, in an effort to promote it and bring in money fast, they offered an annual membership at a very good rate that included free group training as part of the membership. Often, I was the only one in the group or one of only two or three. It was incredible and I learned so much. If finances don't allow, take advantage of what I've learned, try some of the workout videos led by professional trainers, and use the internet. You can find some very inexpensive videos at club and other discount stores for purchase or perhaps access them online.

I belong to 24-hour fitness because they are everywhere, have great classes, and I purchase my membership (two years at a time) very inexpensively at my local Costco. I generally work out three times a week at the gym (twice during the week and once over the weekend) and hike and walk in between but this was a long, slow process for sure. Initially, 15 to 20 minutes of a 50-minute gym class, at say 60%, was as far as I got. Listen to your body and modify and take breaks as needed but just don't quit (or leave) until you've reached whatever commitment you've made for yourself. And, of course, please be realistic!

My favorite gym classes are: body pump, boot camp, cycle (spin), and sand bell (a weighted bag class). Although I have some great exercise equipment at home, I rarely use it, as I do better with a structured group setting. I regularly walk to Starbuck's, the market for just a few items, and to the old town section of my city for a variety of things. I also try to do a dinner and hike date with my mother as often as possible; she loves to hike as well and it allows us a little mother daughter time together. Believe it or not, I can't wait for retirement when I can do more.

Exercise, in some form, is vital for me. Please don't misunderstand, you should be able to lose the weight and improve your health by changing the way that you eat alone but there is something so transforming about exercise that I beg you to give it a try. Give it at least 30 days and plenty of experimentation.

10

WORKOUT

"20 percent of adults meet the Physical Activity Guidelines for both aerobic and muscle-strengthening activity," the CDC states.

As always, start where you are but start working out! This can be done at the gym or at home, indoors or outdoors, and with or without equipment. All of my workouts can be modified quite easily to better suit your current level or perhaps minor injuries you may have along the way. For what it's worth, I have experienced a tiny tear in the meniscus, nerve damage to the bottom of my feet, as well as a neck and back injury from a car accident in late 2014. After physical therapy, chiropractic care, and massage I am in better condition than before the injuries. In my experience, exercise is always a healthy part of recovery.

Here are some routines you may want to experiment with:

Routine #1

50 jumping jacks (or jump rope)

40 squats (traditional, narrow leg, wide leg)

30 abs (traditional sit ups, crunches with feet in air, bicycles, crunches on ball, etc.)

20 biceps (10 each arm)

10 push ups

Routine #2

100 jumping jacks (or jump rope)

75 squats (traditional, narrow leg, wide leg)

50 lunges (25 each leg)

25 bridge (for 25 seconds)

Routine #3

100 jumping jacks (or jump rope)

90 squats (traditional, narrow leg, wide leg)

80 lunges (40 each leg - stationary or walking)

70 leg lifts (35 each leg)

60 pelvic thrusts

50 bend over on one leg (25 each leg)

40 biceps (20 each arm)

30 bridge (for 30 seconds)

20 calf raises

10 push ups

Switch out anything you like or change the order. There are so many different variations of arm, leg and ab exercises that you could use these three routines for life. You can also do the third routine, that goes from 100 down to 10, counting by 20's rather than 10's. When it comes to arms, you can either use hand held weights, that you can purchase pretty inexpensively, or things that you have around the house. Whatever you do, don't wait to get the right equipment. Canned vegetables, or something along those lines, will work just fine to start.

Again, if this looks like way too much, modify! Try starting at 25 and moving down by 5. Choose simpler options. Try marching in place, push-ups against the wall, and perhaps some arm exercises without any weight.

11

COMMITMENT

"If you are persistent you will get it, if you are consistent you will keep it." Jeromy Shingongo.

I believe in NO MATTER WHAT'S. They work. I can't have a cheat day once in a while so I don't do it EVER. I have cut certain things out of my diet and I don't eat them no matter what. I also exercise regularly no matter what. Again, I don't eat wheat, flour, or sugar and I have three weekly classes at the gym and walk and hike in between.

That being said, starting out was a little brutal. Detoxing from all the chemicals and preservatives, not to mention caffeine, was pretty awful. The good news is you only have to do it once if you cut them out completely. You can end that vicious cycle of craving, binging, and detoxing, not to mention all the latest diets, by not putting those substances into your system NO MATTER

WHAT.

Most importantly for me, when it's time to eat, please eat NO MATTER WHAT. Don't let anything come before your abstinence - not even your husband or children because you won't be of much use to them if you're lost in the vicious cycle of food addiction. So, eat what you need to when you need to NO MATTER WHAT.

When it comes to exercise, I recommend small goals and slowly working your way up. Again, I was lucky to do one third of a gym class when I first got started. Listen to your body, and modify and take breaks as needed, but, just don't quit (or leave) until you've reached whatever commitment you've made to yourself NO MATTER WHAT.

I did a lot of using 15-minute increments and only increased the time after several weeks of doing the same class. Perhaps 15 minutes the first month, 30 minutes the second month, and essentially the entire class by the third month but, if you have to do it 5 minutes at a time, do that NO MATTER WHAT. Cycle (spin class), part of my regiment today, had to be 5 minutes at a time and it's still a real accomplishment when I make it through the entire class.

Most instructors will offer modifications but don't hesitate to request them if they don't. When dealing with injuries, and limitations, be sure to tell the instructor. They are generally really wonderful about that kind of thing. You may even receive a little extra attention which won't hurt your cause at all. Occasionally, instructors can be a little touchy about members doing their own thing during class or leaving early but if you let them know you can generally avoid that kind of awkwardness.

There have been times where I was incredibly busy, working two jobs and going back to school, for instance. Also, although generally pretty healthy, I have been sick. Despite these challenges my food has remained clean and I have exercised to whatever extent my body allowed, again NO MATTER WHAT.

I keep chicken broth in the freezer. Clean chicken soup can be made with shredded chicken, any vegetables, and 1 cup of brown rice. If you don't have the chicken on hand throw two eggs and bring it to a boil on the stove (and then add the rice). Clean smoothies can be a life saver too, when you have the flu, for instance.

I vividly recall having food poisoning last year. My mother and a dear friend took turns coming by to take care of me. They heated up broth, made me smoothies, picked up and delivered a couple things that are easier to digest, and prepared whatever I thought I could stomach while they were here.

As I mentioned, I have also had a few injuries along the way and some were a bit debilitating. While I was forced to modify quite a bit, I nevertheless found a way to do what I could safely. There have been times where I could only do upper body or lower body, for a period of time, and others where I could perhaps do some light walking but was in no condition to do my usual 5.7-mile hike.

There were, of course, times where I had to take a break because I was in bed for several days but I always got right back to whatever my body allowed; it really is part of getting better. Working my way back up to my normal regimen has sometimes been a slow and tedious process but it is so worth it. See the doctor, take advantage of physical therapy (do the exercises they give you) and use a brace if necessary.

So, COMMITMENT to your health, to yourself, and your routine is essential. Structure is huge so make a schedule, ideally attending the same classes (or whatever) every week. I go to a weighted bag class Sunday morning, a boot camp Monday evening, and cycle (spin) Wednesday or Thursday depending on my schedule. I try to hike with my mom on Tuesday, Wednesday, or Thursday depending on our schedules. I still love Starbucks (even black decaf) and like to pick up fresh produce from the market so I walk regularly to both, as well.

12

BE KIND TO YOURSELF

"Self-care is never a selfish act - it is simply good stewardship of the only gift I have, the gift I was put on earth to offer to others." Parker Palmer

Understanding that this should probably be the first chapter, it came to me now, and I felt inspired to end with it. Food addiction (binging, purging, starving, detoxing, etc.) is a lonely, nasty, painful business. We abuse our bodies, and our psyches, so terribly; so, please be kind to yourself. Take bubble baths or walks for pleasure, drink clean tea or bubbly water, journal or talk to a close friend. When you can't get it all in, take care of you first. Contrary to popular belief, it is not selfish and will make you more useful (and pleasant) to everyone around you.

Find a way to reward yourself. It doesn't have to be

terribly expensive; it may not have a monetary value at all. I can't seem to remember what it was but I rewarded myself with something special when I reached 30 days of abstinence. Then, when I really started dropping weight, I bought myself a new pair of pants every time I went down a size. I remember buying inexpensive jeans from Costco and how great it was when they didn't fit anymore. Eventually, things started falling off me, literally.

I don't make much money but I have found a couple of high-end consignment shops where I can afford to get the brands and styles I want for a fraction of the price. Ironically, I dress better than I ever have and spend significantly less money on clothing. I recently got a really cute skirt at Target on clearance for $6.00 and I get so many compliments every time I wear it. My gym sells name brand workout wear, and regularly clearances things out, and at the holidays marks everything down by 40%. I just got two pairs of my favorite Nike workout pants for $27 each.

Some of the things I have rewarded myself with over time (and asked for as gifts as well by the way) are actually for exercise. I got myself a very nice Pilates mat, cycle shoes (for spin class), and a hot pink Bosu ball. I have also received workout clothes, equipment, and my favorite hiking shoes as gifts.

The only thing I might caution you about is treating yourself with food. Although, going to a more expensive healthy restaurant, or over-priced market, or even just spending way too much on expensive water is certainly fine, treating yourself with food can be a very sneaky business, as most of us have some deeply engrained old ideas that can continue to work on our consciousness, even when we don't realize it.

Again, be kind to yourself.

My Story

My relationship with food was unhealthy from the very start. I never seemed to have an off switch. Ironically, I was so thin growing up, and a bit athletic, that my over-eating was almost encouraged. I have memories of competing with my dad and brother at the dinner table to see who could eat the most food. I remember vividly sitting in front of the chips and dip at the holidays and eating until I was sick. It was a running joke in my family. I would eat *all* the onion dip and then scrape the pan of mom's scalloped potatoes at meal time.

Although my mother is a wonderful cook, she was working and going to school for a good deal of my childhood. Consequently, we ate a lot of casual, fast, junk food. Mom would make hamburger patties and then slather them in canned chili and American cheese, hotdogs wrapped in cheese and crescent dough, and we ate a lot of boxed macaroni and cheese (sometimes mom added canned tuna and then it was tuna casserole).

Although we didn't eat particularly healthy growing up, we never seemed to have the most popular goodies, and typical junk food, that my friends had in the house and I was always looking for a way to get it. I went to church with my childhood girlfriend's family every chance I got, for instance, and snuck out to buy junk food at the liquor store with the money mom gave me for church offering. I also recall going to Magic Mountain on a school field trip and spending all the money mom gave me (including what I was supposed to use to buy my little brother something) on junk food.

I did a lot of babysitting when I was still quite young and frequently would eat all the junk food in their house and then be embarrassed about it. I remember one time when I opened a brand-new box of pop tarts and ate not one package (two pop tarts) but two and then was so worried about what they would think of me that I hid the rest in my bag, hoping that it would be overlooked.

Then, no surprise, I ended up eating the last package as well. I recall realizing years later that I had stolen from my neighbor, in order to satisfy a craving that seemed beyond my control. Today, I believe that it was; I know that food addiction is real.

If you relate to this at all, I would really encourage you to read Kay Sheppard's, *From The First Bite*. As I mentioned in my acknowledgments, her understanding of food addiction and work in the field saved my life. Although it was passed on to me with some minor adjustments, her food plan is the basis for how I eat today.

I am so passionate about food today that the people in my life get a kick out of it. I get excited about clean food and cooking. I took pictures of my food, long before I started posting it. I love the way food looks, smells, and tastes. I love the presentation on a plate. I love planning meals and shopping for the ingredients. I love all the colors. And, of course, I love eating!

I eat so good that sometimes it feels like I get to splurge without any of the awful consequences. I can eat delicious food, until I feel almost gorged with certain meals, and still lose or maintain my weight, and feel incredible. I also have meals that feel significantly lighter that I can enjoy before a workout, over the summer, or when I'm a little under the weather physically.

Most importantly, I have a kind of freedom from food today that I've never had, and in fact didn't even know existed. I no longer feel ruled by food and my addiction to it. I have found that exercise not only supports that but changes your body in ways that eating right alone cannot. I'm more grateful than I know how to say that I feel as fit as I do mentally and physically. My life is well-rounded and whole in a way that is indescribably wonderful. I really am happier and healthier than I've ever been.

I want to wish you the very best on your journey. My hope is that something I've written will help somewhere along the way. Sharing my experience certainly helps me so thank you for allowing me to share it with you.

Made in the USA
Monee, IL
12 August 2020

38265653R10039